your spirit of purpose, of leadership, and team value are

Change Your Mind,
Change Your Body,
Change Your Life

an inspiration to those you lead. Thank you

Ann Myers RPN BA

for your support throughout the years.

Ann Myers

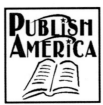

PublishAmerica
Baltimore

First printing

At the specific preference of the author, PublishAmerica allowed this work to remain exactly as the author intended, verbatim, without editorial input.

ISBN: 1-4241-3998-8
PUBLISHED BY PUBLISHAMERICA, LLLP
www.publishamerica.com
Baltimore

Printed in the United States of America

For: Don, my husband, the love of my life, and my best friend. Your integrity lights our path.

Inspired by:

Adam's strength, Andrew's soul, Jonathan's perseverance, Ross' loyalty, Nicholas' athletic skill, Kim Newhook's innate beauty, Joan's talent, Linda's gusto, Mark's quiet dignity, and Bill & Alice's generosity.

Change Your Mind, Change Your Body, Change Your Life

Introduction

Living a life that you love is possible. You can feel sexier, feel more joy, love, happiness, and fulfillment. This book consists of a series of exercises and information that can help you get more of what you really want from life. You are here on this planet at this time for a reason. Not only do you have needs, wants, and dreams you have a purpose. With some determination and a little perseverance, you will unravel the mystery that lies within you and reveal your core truth.

Through this course I want you to be your own best friend, to love yourself, and be fully present for yourself. No more will you ignore your body and pretend that you do not exist. Neither will you abuse your body in order to feel alive. Still the pendulum and find your middle ground between nihilism and rape. Make love to yourself. Approve of yourself. Be your own best friend.

Read this book in any order that feels comfortable to you. Take what feels right and dismiss the rest. This book is a tool for you to use. You are a miracle and only you know what is best for you.

"Treading a Way does not consist in mechanically applying a technique until liberation is achieved. There are no magic formulas or assembly-line techniques. Each person must come up with his or her own Way-by giving up most dearly held convictions and habits, by making use of all resources, by doing the most extraordinary spiritual somersault."
Piero Ferrucci

Making Miracles Happen

The Ideal Body at Any Age

Is yours! Never mind what you have learned in the past to think what an ideal body is. Eradicate notions of skinny and young as being the ideal. You are not stuck. You have the power to live fully in the gorgeous, lean, exciting machine that the Universe is lending to you right now.

As children the adults surrounding us often invalidated our emotions. "You aren't hungry, you just ate!" " That's nothing to be sad about." "Don't be angry." On top of that we were fed a diet of negative beliefs about ourselves. "You're a waste of time, you can't do that." "You're too small." "You're too big." "You're not smart enough." "You are lazy." "You are hyperactive." Growing up feeling useless and trapped creates beliefs of powerlessness and hopelessness.

Emotions like shame and fear overwhelm us and direct our actions and our actions define our lives. However, it is our thoughts that fuel our emotions. If we can nourish ourselves with good, healthy food, and clean water, it follows that we can nourish ourselves with good, clean, healthy thoughts.

Every thought we have manifests itself in our perceptions of our bodies, our environment, and ourselves. Our thoughts become our reality. The only person thinking in our heads is us therefore we have control over our experience of reality.

"Realize that the journey to the center takes place within your own mind."

Mathew Flickstein, Journey to the Center.

Take Care of Your Body
by Using Your Mind

Here is an exercise that is designed to clear your brain and body of negative labels and reprogram it with vibrancy.

1. Develop a list of words that describe your best possible body. Use a thesaurus or dictionary to get some ideas. Taut, streamlined, healthy, fresh, vigorous, energetic, gorgeous, beautiful, dynamic, luminous, spectacular, unique, vibrant, glorious, regal, lithe, muscular, flexible.
2. Make "I am" statements using your name, for example: "I Ann, am lithe, healthy, flexible, dynamic, and energized."
3. Now squeeze and flex your gluteus maximus (butt) muscles as tightly as you can.
4. Then release.
5. As you are doing this, in rhythmic cadence repeat your affirmations for your ideal body.
6. I am a vigorous, sexy, lean, healthy, human being.
7. I am unique and spectacular.
8. Remember to use your name and to use the present tense. Because you already are fabulous!
9. Breathe long and soft and love yourself.
10. Repeat this exercise often throughout the day.

Your Natural State is Grace

"There is always a certain peace in being what one is, in being that completely."
Ugo Betti.

You may have been raised to believe that you can have it all and be anything you want to be and while this is true there are some who believe that they have to be everything to everyone just to be acceptable. It may be time to slow down and figure out what turns you on. What makes you happy? What can you do to make yourself happy? You do not need to be on display. Try to focus on yourself as the subject of your life not as an object in someone else's life.

"Create the kind of self you will be happy to live with all of your life."
Foster C. McClelland

Definition of Success

Developing your definition of success is a necessary step in creating a life that you love to live. However, before you can define success you need to know who you are. When you know who you are you will also know what makes you happy. The following are some of the questions that you can ask yourself that will help you on your self-awareness journey.

- What is the main focus in your life? Is it your family, your love life, your relationships, your career, your health, or your finances?
- Would your focus change if your life were in balance?
- Emotionally are you interested in becoming more assertive, less fearful, more peaceful, more confident, less angry, or more secure?
- In relationships are you dominant, submissive, needy, or demanding?
- Do you want to be more dependent or more independent?
- Do you consider interdependence an option for you?
- What were you raised to believe about the world?
- Is it safe or unsafe to trust others?
- Are ethics important to you?
- Do you want to have more integrity?
- Can you be honest with yourself?
- Were you abused growing up?
- Are you abusive to yourself or others?

Next you look at what you like about yourself. List everything about yourself that you like. Don't worry if you can't think of anything right now because by the end of the course you'll have lots to like about yourself.

The next few questions can help you get an idea of what you find joyful.

- What did you like to do as a child?
- What did you do as a teenager that was fun and healthy?
- What engaged, enthralled, and absorbed your attention? List every-thing from that time.
- List everything that you like to do now.

Take some time right now to write down everything that you want to be, what you want more of from life, and anything that is working well right now but you maybe are afraid of losing.

Take your desires and put them into present tense, positive self-statements. For example, "I am healthy, intelligent, and wealthy." This is the beginning of your definition of success.

Now you get to write down everything you don't like about yourself. Put it down on paper, mark it, "for my eyes-only" if you want but do write down everything that you want to change about yourself and your life. All of your negative traits, beliefs, actions, and the things that you want to stop doing or believing. The things that cause you pain. Some of the things that cause you pain might be acceptable to you if you could control them. Things like drugs, alcohol, and relationships. These things are not so straightforward but they are looked at in detail in subsequent chapters.

Everything that you have written down about yourself that you would like to change has served a purpose in your life. It is however, time to challenge your coping strategies. So, can you flip the negative and make it a positive? If so, do it. Maybe it is something that you have to eradicate altogether, therefore, create a statement that does not include the problem. For example, "I can handle anything with healthy coping strategies."

You may need a therapist to work with you through your personal inventory. Not only can a therapist give you support for the emotional pain that comes up when you work on your issues but a therapist can also guide you through self-deception toward a clear understanding of your truth.

Once you have a good grasp of who and what you are, and who and what you would like to be, you can begin the task of designing your own self-statements. To design your definition of success think about what success feels like to you. It can be joy, warmth, respect, integrity, strength, health, love, security, and freedom. Next figure out what success looks like to you. Is it numerous friends, a few close friends, a best friend, wealth, invitations, a beautiful home, luxury vehicle, travel, everything that you could ever need or want? Or is it time to do the things that you have always wanted to do, time to reflect, time to share your gifts?

Take some time now and fully develop and then write down your definition of success. Other ways to view it are as a personal mission statement or what success means to you. Make sure it is positive, in the first person, and that you already have it. Post your definition in a place where you can see it often. Memorize it and repeat it to yourself throughout the day. Use it as a mantra to help you sleep at night.

My own definition of success has changed throughout my life. Right now my definition of success is, "I live my life with integrity. I recognize and respect the divine light in every person that I meet. I facilitate joy, prosperity, and peace. My family is safe, happy, and successful."

"Many of life's failures are people who did not realize how close they were to success when they gave up."
  Thomas Edison

The Flame

Cloaked in mystery, meditation was touted as the new age spiritual messiah and a magical cure-all for western society. Meditation isn't a quick fix or a cure-all but it is a powerful tool for cleansing, healing, and soothing the mind, soul, and spirit. You will need to make a quiet, alone space for yourself that is comfortable and conducive to relaxation but not sleep. It is best done in an upright manner with open palms upward gently resting on the knees. Seated in a chair is fine. You can lay down in a comfortable position. The only problem with that though is that you may fall asleep. Meditation occurs when the gamma waves of your brain begin a rhythmic cycle. During this wave pattern you can manifest your thoughts with the most productivity and clarity. So you can begin by learning to meditate and then choose to do your positive affirmations when you are clear and clean in the gamma rhythm.

To begin you sit in position. Open and relaxed. Close your eyes. Concentrate on the flow of oxygen and air that you draw in through your nostrils, hold deeply and gently in your lungs. Then a long exhale out through your mouth. Visualize the air moving in a complete circle in through your nose, around through your lungs, and out through your mouth. Quietly still your mind. In the velvet soft blackness in your mind picture a single, glowing, flickering flame. Concentrate all your focus and thought on this golden, flickering, luminescent light. Allow thoughts to come and go without any attachment. Wish them well and let them be on their way. Continue to focus on the soft, black, inner backdrop of your mind with the single luminescent, flickering light, licking, lightly, gently, and glowing.

Practice meditation daily preferably at sunrise. Relax, surrender yourself, and succumb to joy.

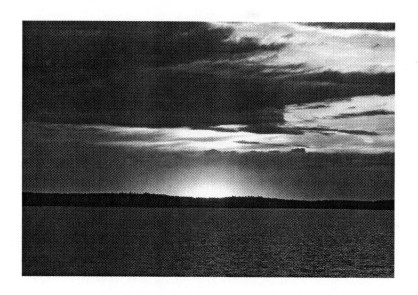

"You are a system of Light, as are all beings. The frequency of your Light depends upon your consciousness. When you shift the level of your consciousness, you shift the frequency of your Light."
Gary Zukav

Intangible Planes

In all of existence there is but one power. In all of life there is a

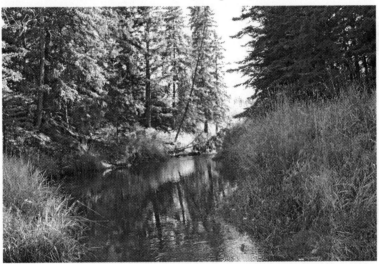

golden presence of joy. How then do we exploit this creation, this joy? How can we achieve happiness?

Our thoughts trigger our emotions and joy and bliss are emotional characteristics. Often our emotions direct our behaviors. Actions and behaviors are strong leaders of personal reality because actions and behaviors lead the individual's direction in life. We need to monitor our thoughts, address the results of our thinking, and accept our accountability for our experience. Our actions can be corrected. Our detrimental physical habits need to be corrected because the secret to health, longevity, and peace lie in the physical realm. Our bodies nourish our brains and a healthy brain thinks better than a tired, poisoned, or malnourished brain.

Thought is the highest form of change and cleanliness to be attained. Also the most difficult. When there is thought a web of energy moves and the resulting action transmutes into goal. What is our thought becomes our reality. Unseen molecular energy is constantly fluctuating and gathering momentum. In magical sequence you get exactly what you believe that you have in real time. What you experience as the present moment. Fear and anger act as a lightning rod to dust and can powerfully and instantaneously give results. Also does love, joy, and orgasmic energy. Powerful emotions and physical activity create ideal conditions for results, as does meditation when the brain is in a high-frequency gamma wave pattern.

In order to clearly manifest your desires you first need behavioral integrity. Be honest, scrupulously truthful with yourself. Give freely with joy. Let go of all negativity. Forgive, forgive, forgive! Yourself and all others. Forgive the universe. Embrace truth, integrity, love, and trust that you are whole, complete, and invaluable to existence. Once you are clean with yourself, no stealing, no lying, no dubious behavior, absolutely honest with yourself, then you can begin to delve within. Ask what is it that would bring you the greatest joy? What do you need to be happy? Wealth? Good food? Sunshine? Love? Acknowledged as being special? Creative expression? Health? Freedom?

Then be specific, be in present tense, be exact, be fully involved and utilize meditation, physical activity, and loving emotions to think your positive reality. Then trust your instincts and act on what the universe presents.

Do You Want to Change?

A desire to change is the key component. Once you have desire, the energy to move towards the goal, that is the electricity, the magic that sets all the wheels in motion. Desire attracts itself back and thus the ten-fold rule stands true. That is you get back ten times what you give out. Desire acts as a magnet to change agents drawing them from numerous sources. You need only express your desire, that what you wish. Whisper it into the vast subconscious realm, couple it with your desire to change and voila you have the magic recipe. Alchemy instantaneously. Miracles can and do happen. If you are unsure of the process you can try it for a game, jokingly, but use true intent. Pick a tangible object, big or small, expensive, rare, or cheap and common. Pick it on a whim. I picked a, "dozen red roses on my television set". I became disillusioned when I didn't get any roses but then I noticed that every time I watched T.V. I saw a dozen red roses. I then changed my affirmation to, "I have a dozen roses **on top of** my TV" and bingo! within a few days roses arrived, unsolicited by me. See it, believe it, own it, and know it in the present tense. Repeatedly mantra your desire in thought form. Dance it gracefully through your brain and when it manifests you will be enthralled in process. It is a totally fun game. Once you are confident that it can work for you create a mantra that states who you are with the change that you want. For example, "I am honest, I have integrity." The real magic begins when you use this in service to others. You open your energy to giving that what others need.

You can use your spiritual resources to guide, give information, lend a hand, heal with touch, or heal with a perfect word. Service is the most rewarding fun of all.

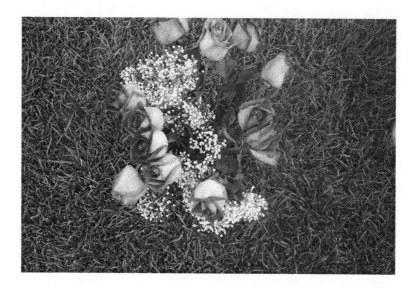

Life of Service

Why should we live a life of service? What's in it for me you might ask? The light and glow that grows within the soul of another human being that can be switched on with love and witnessed by others heals all who can sense it. We all have the power to ignite joy in the soul of another. It is effortless and increases the energy of the igniter.

How do you do this? You live fully for yourself. You meet all of your own needs and find your own safety within yourself. Then when you meet others you come from a place of comfort and strength that can recognize this in the other. It is on a spiritual level that this recognition takes place. You seek competence in the other and find the internal rightness. It is always there. You facilitate an environment where the best in others is safe to show. You smile, look directly into their eyes. You take an open body posture. Your attitude is to give. Energy emanates freely from your center outward in all directions from your body. Because you have no expectation of reciprocation it doesn't matter what the other does with your kindness.

It is at its most simple an attitude of acceptance that others are doing the best that they can with what they have been given. It is non-judgmental. It is empathy without pity. It is non-sexual and needs no physical expression. You can do it in any relationship and in any field of employment.

Because energy is infinite, neither created nor destroyed, you have an internal endless ability to give it out. You need only be a conduit or channel. So all the principles of taking care of you apply. You need a healthy system to most easily be of service.

The only caution that I propose to you is to not be a doormat. Kindness is not weakness. You are autonomous, you can and should say no to inappropriate requests for your kindness. You'll instinctively know when you are being drawn beyond appropriate limits by a gut feeling of wrongness. You'll feel agitated and uncomfortable. Simply stand back and center yourself. It is a bit of a dance with energy. It is give and take but it all takes place within your energy system. The energy is constantly flowing from deep within you to outside of you. Don't try to take energy out of others into yourself. There is a natural exchange of warmth when positive connections are made but don't try to draw energy out of unknown persons.

In a close, trusted, personal relationship energy is more relaxed and free flowing and you can safely absorb from outside of yourself. In an intimate sexual relationship energy commingles. The yoga practice of Tantric sex asserts that when partners approach each other as god and goddess, utilizing open energy chakkras, an unbelievable orgasmic experience is the reward.

A life lived in service to positive energy fields brings tangible and exciting rewards.

Feel it, be it, do it. I think you're going to love it!

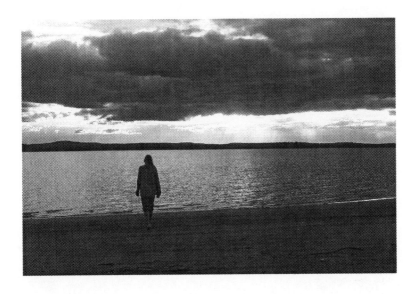

"Mind precedes its objects. They are mind-governed and mind-made. To speak or act with a peaceful mind, is to draw happiness after oneself, like an inseparable shadow."
   Buddha

An Exercise and Challenge
The Human Fast

- Be silent.
- Embrace solitude.
- Eat only nutritious foods.
- Drink lots of clean water.
- No other substances
- Think only positive thoughts, open and upward.
- Stretch and exercise.
- Create.
- Love yourself.
- Radiate love.
- Enjoy safety.
- Embrace joy.
- Be honest.
- Live fully in the present moment.
- Be gentle with yourself and with others.
- Be prosperous.
- Be purposeful.
- Give.
- Love giving.
- Be of service.
- Be humble.
- Be honest.
- Be yourself. Be human.
- Forgive.
- Forget.
- Move on.
- Be thankful
- Do this for one minute.
- Do this for one hour.
- Do this as much as you can.

"We are what we repeatedly do. Excellence, then, is not an act, but a habit."
   Aristotle

The Heart of the Matter

Energy. Pick up a fresh, clean piece of lettuce and a scrubbed chunk of fresh carrot. Really look at them and tune into the energy and vibration they are giving out. You can see it, you can feel it, and you can taste it. It is real and alive. Everything is. Sub atomic particles. Quantum theory. We are swirling, interacting fields of energy. Our vast inner realm of subconscious mind is interconnected with all others in the universe. A storehouse of limitless energy, infinity. Our thoughts are directed energy. We create in every moment.

Exercise and Mantra
Start your day:

Stand up with your feet shoulder width apart. Arms and shoulders relaxed comfortably at your sides. Knees slightly bent (over your toes). Breathing in through your nose reach your arms out and up over your head, bring your arms back down, to your sides while you breathe out through your mouth.

Using your inner voice repeat the following mantra:

I am whole, free, and brand new. I am refreshed, comfortable, and excited. Every moment is new and alive. I am new and alive. I have the power to create and change my own thoughts and beliefs. I am free and spontaneous. I am loving and loved. Kindness matters. I am beautiful from the inside out. I am beautiful from the outside in. I am safe.

You can memorize this mantra (or record it) and then while the mantra runs through your mind, gently move your body, sway and dance to your inner rhythm.

"Of what is the body made? It is made of emptiness and rhythm. At the ultimate heart of the world, there is no solidarity. Once again, there is only the dance."
George Leonard

Distracting Yourself

Preventing Self-harm behavior

Borderline Personality Disorder is a diagnosis that is often given to people who struggle emotionally and have feelings of low self-worth. Symptoms of the disorder are discordant personal relationships, emotional deregulation with rapid mood swings of volatile anger, irritability, and sadness, unpredictable behavior, self-mutilation, and suicidal ideation.

The cause is not straightforward; however, people who were raised in an environment where feelings were not validated and bodies were abused are often diagnosed with Borderline Personality Disorder.

If ever your emotions are so out of control that you are at risk of hurting yourself, use any of these techniques to distract yourself:

- Watch a movie.
- Go for a walk.
- Punch a pillow.
- Take a piece of ice and hold it in your hand and feel it melt, let your anger and pain flow and melt out with the ice.
- Meditate using positive affirmations repeatedly. Put your favorite one on the next line.

- Close your eyes and breathe deeply five times in a row.
- Contact someone who cares about you.
- Call a crisis line.
- Exercise and Mantra

Stand up tall and strong. Tense your body then relax. Breathe out as you tense and breathe in as you relax. Tense and relax.

Repeat: I am a child of the Universe. I am one with the Universe that created me. I am intact, glorious, and free. I am special. I love myself. I am complete. I own my life, my feelings, my mind, my body, and my choices. I am in control of myself. I trust my love. I trust myself. I trust my feelings and intuitions. I am strong and free. I am unique and special. I like myself. I appreciate myself. I accept myself.

The after effects of abuse can cause you to be emotionally volatile. This results in self-defeating behavior and the cycle of destruction continues. When you begin to monitor and control your thoughts you will discover that you are also monitoring and controlling your emotions. Make controlling your self-harm impulses your goal, commit to your goal and trust that the Universe that created you loves you and wants only for you to be happy and safe.

Practice Forgiveness

When you choose to forgive it does not mean that you are agreeing with the wrong that has been done. You are not condoning abusive behavior. You forgive in order to release yourself from the hold that the injury or the perpetrator has over you. Revenge may be sweet but forgiveness is salvation.

"Overcome anger by love, evil by good, overcome the miser by giving, overcome the liar by truth."
Buddha

This is in no way intended to minimize the overwhelming pain that people suffer when their lives are torn by intentional harm. It is simply that forgiveness is a gift that you give to yourself. Practicing forgiveness will take you through waves of resentment, blame, anger, and hurt until you eventually feel light with grace.

Visualization Exercise:

Close your eyes and breathe deeply for a count of ten. Picture in your mind the event or person that needs forgiveness. Imagine that there is a thin, wispy line attaching you to this object of forgiveness. Now imagine that there is a large, golden pair of scissors that cleanly cuts the line and as the object floats away and disappears repeat to yourself, "I forgive you, I let you go, go in peace, I am free." Imagine yourself bathed in golden light.

When you are able to release painful blocks through forgiveness you will be free to move on.

"It isn't the mountain ahead that wears you out-it's the grain of sand in your shoe."
Robert Service

Make an Area in Your Home
Your Special Area

Take a mat, cushions, blanket, comforter, candle, table, comfortable chair, a place to write, room to stretch out and lay down, and enough room to move freely about. Take meaningful items to your special place. Make it yours over time, no need to rush or clutter it. Create a comfortable personal space just for you. Perhaps a C.D. player or an audio player with ocean waves, forest sounds, or peaceful music.

You can use your area for anything that you want. Maybe you would like to draw or paint? You could journal, write poetry, sing, meditate, or dance.

Try this exercise to help you feel comfortable in the freedom and safety of your own space:

1) At a minimum you'll need a piece of paper and a pencil. If you have watercolors, pastels, or colors of any kind, you can use them for this challenge.
2) Draw a picture of your higher self and your definition of success. That is, a picture of your most spiritually developed form of you in a scene that illustrates you living successfully. If it will help you can use words. Once you are finished put your picture up to remind yourself of your highest ideal.

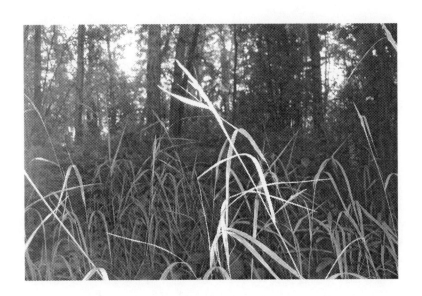

Breathing

Taking deep breaths that expand the chest wall produces instantaneous relaxation. The combination of increased oxygen and stretched thoracic muscles is a universal signal to the body that it is o.k. to relax. Draw a deep, slow breath in through the nostrils holding for two seconds in the lungs, then release slowly through a relaxed open mouth. Your exhale should be almost twice as long as your inhale. Slow, circular, deep, expanding, rolling breaths.

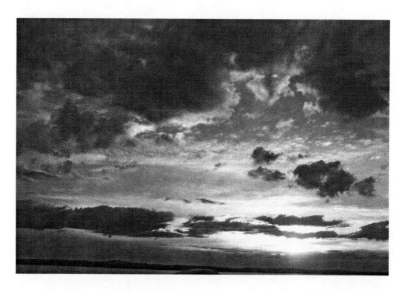

At any stressful moment simply close your eyes and breathe in slowly, relaxing your stomach, hold your breath deeply in your lower lungs for four seconds then gently release. This helps to train you to have an internal locus of control because it instantly connects you to your inner process. Deep breathing combats stress and stress-related illness. It also expels toxins and burns calories.

Healing Breath

The universe breathes pure, clean, light through me and of me. All is infinity, peaceful, and right. In the endless circle of life I am centered, perfect, and complete. Essence of purity cleanses through me with every circular breath. Inhalation of fresh, cool, moist, prana, exhalation out, ever gentle always relaxed, letting go, releasing. Circular intake of perfect air, prana, life, the universe itself glides suffusing through permeating every pore with health, washing with freedom, peace, love, forgiveness. Angelic sweeps of ever lifting gentle swirls of peace and love and kindness. Beauty and transcendence glide and lift me heavenward on clouds of joy. Pure radiant, golden light inside me glowing warm and healing. Coursing through my veins, flooding joy, blissful, gorgeous freedom. Truth, beauty, love it's all that matters. Exquisite radiant light emanates from within. Translucent beauty, liquid light, shining, glowing, healthy. Transforming every molecule into health and joy. Lightness and perfection. Sweetness and grace. Falling into myself, I fall in love with myself. I am in love with my magnificence, my power to create with love, beauty, and joy. The universe breathes through me. I am translucent light. Capture all the beauty I possess and inhale fully then slowly let beauty and grace flow out and around and surround me. Circling in with a full, fresh inhalation of exquisite lightness, perfect love. Magically light I lift from within and attune to my vast infinite nature. Plunging inward I see beauty, love, truth, grace, kindness. Floating inward, gently gliding I see crystalline, purity, clarity of thought, fountains of creativity, an abundance of wealth, and beauty. I am gorgeous, beautiful, one with the universe that created me. Always gracious, centered, and controlled.

Channeling Energy

The nicest and possibly easiest way to ready yourself for channeling power is to treat your physical body as well as you possibly can. Feed it the healthiest, most nutritious food that you can find. If you can grow your own vegetables or sprouts, do so. Otherwise pick the most vibrant, colorful fruit, and vegetables from the store. Colorful fruits, vegetables, and beans contain phytochemicals and antioxidants. When you eat these healthy nutrients you combat cancer and aging. Wash produce thoroughly to remove the pesticides that are sprayed on them while they are growing. A healthy option is to buy organically grown produce. Prepare vegetables with the least amount of destruction possible. Gently steam as opposed to boiling.

Don't use styrofoam or plastic wrap in the microwave because they breakdown and the chemicals are released into your food. Instead use porcelain or glass. Avoid partially-hydrogenated fat, a.k.a. transfatty acids. Don't eat burnt fat or burnt protein.

Eat omega 3, 6, 7, and 9 fatty acids; omega 3 is found in flaxseeds, soya beans, and fatty fish like salmon, mackeral, and anchovies. Omegas 6 and 9 are in vegetable oils. Omega 7 is found in macadamia nuts. Look for Omega-3 enriched foods. Chickens that are fed flaxseeds produce omega-3 enriched eggs. Try drinking soy milk, eating tofu, edame beans, and soya nuts to up your intake of omega 3 fatty acids and, especially for women over forty, to get isoflavanoids which help regulate hormones.

Drink fresh, clean water and lots of it. At least 6-8 ounce glasses daily; the water in non-caffeinated and non-alcoholic beverages counts toward your total intake. In North America tap water should be fine but you do have the option to drink reverse osmosis, purified, or boiled and filtered water.

Avoid simple carbohydrates such as white bread, white sugar, cookies, donuts, and candy. Do eat complex carbohydrates such as fruits, vegetables, and grains. Choose whole grains and unprocessed foods as close to nature as possible. Rolled oats, bran, wheat germ, whole wheat, lentils, beans, almonds, cashews, sunflower seeds, sesame seeds, prunes, and bananas are all great foods.

You also need lean protein to build and repair your body. High quality protein should be eaten 2-3 times per day. Try to eat fish as often as possible but limit tuna to once per week because tuna has been found to have a high mercury content. Only eat wild salmon because farmed salmon is high in toxic chemicals.

Eat calcium rich foods to assist with weight loss. Foods high in calcium include milk, yogurt, cheese, (choose the low fat varieties), tinned salmon (you have to eat the bones), spinach, and broccoli. By increasing your calcium intake you are also combating osteoporosis.

Diet

The number of calories that you need in a day depends on your height, weight, activity level, and metabolism. To get an approximate calorie quota take your ideal weight and multiply it by 10. This is the amount of calories you would burn if you rested all day. When you are exercising moderately multiply your ideal body weight by 12 and that is the number of calories you can consume to reach and maintain your goal weight.

- Drink at least 6-8 glasses of water a day.
- Eat the skins and seeds of fruit and vegetables when possible.
- Limit salt, caffeine, and alcohol.
- Avoid aspartame and use the sweetener stevia instead.
- Soy is a good source of protein.
- Egg-whites are protein with zero fat.
- Dark chocolate improves your mood.
- Dry red wine, in moderation, is good for you.
- Supplement with calcium citrate because it is absorbed through the intestinal cells and between the cells as well. Therefore its' bioavailability is higher than other forms of calcium.
- Drink green tea to increase your intake of polyphenols and antioxidants.
- Eat small meals approximately 5 times a day.
- Fish oils are brain food. If you use a fish oil supplement make sure

it has been molecularly distilled to eliminate mercury, PCB's, and other toxins.
- To combat macular degeneration supplement your diet with zinc, lutein, zeaxanthin, and vitamins A (in the form of beta-caratene), C, and E.
- Flax seeds, sesame seeds, and soy stabilize hormones and have anti-cancer effects.
- Try eating sea vegetables such as kelp, spirulina, and dulce, to assist with weight loss and improve your immune system.
- Greens + multi is an excellent product that has been proven to in-crease physical and mental health.

Live a Long and Healthy Life

In 1976 Dr. Makoto Suzuki and his team of researchers began studying the centenarians (people who are a hundred-years-old and older) of Okinawa, Japan. The researchers were looking for clues as to why these people were so energetic, healthy, slim, and had the greatest longevity in the world.

The team found that the Okinawan diet is low-calorie, low-fat, and high in complex carbohydrates. They eat up to twenty servings a day of fruits and vegetables. They eat fish, soy, dark, green sea-vegetables, sweet potatoes, fruits, onions, green peppers, bean sprouts, rice, bread, and very little poultry, eggs or meat.

They also:

- Drink alcohol in moderation. (Two drinks or less per day).
- Have strong family and community ties.
- Are active throughout the day.
- Maintain rituals that include dancing and Tai Chi.

An article released on August 31, 2004, by Dr. Bradley Wilcox, a member of the Okinawan research team, identified that calorie

44

reduction (1,900 calories per day for men) leads to a longer life. Animal studies corroborate Drs. Suzukis' and Wilcoxs' findings.

"The most important dietary rule for longevity is systematic undereating."
Dan Millman

I attract the perfect vitamins, minerals, and nutrients to me that nourish, repair, and revitalize my system. I honor my health and my body.

Getting to Know Your Body

In order to stretch, lengthen, and relax your muscles you have to get to know them. So, lay flat on the floor and rhythmically clench and release each muscle group starting from your toes, through ankles, calves, knees, quads, buttocks, inner thighs, abdominals, small of back, chest, diaghram, shoulders, middle back, neck, biceps, lower arms, and hands. Simply relax and let loose all your face muscles. Fully relax your body. Now, do this again concentrating on breathing through each body part, muscle group as you gently tense and release. Concentrate on prana, in and out, breathing, warming each muscle, cleaning each fiber and cell, relaxing, and healing. Try to breathe from your belly. Place one hand on your chest and the other hand on your abdomen. When you breathe in and out the hand on your abdomen should move up and down more than the hand on your chest. Once you have run through your whole body with breath, stand up with feet shoulder-width apart and stretch your arms out gently up and out and breathe in fully, then relax. While continuing to stand isometrically tense and relax each muscle, or each muscle group with healthy cleansing, healing breath. Start with your feet by standing gently, rolling onto the balls of your feet to tense calf muscles, then relax and stand down. Tense and release your whole body while imagining an iridescent, luminescent, warming, glowing, ultraviolet light. Suffusing your breath and surrounding you totally in its healing power. All your body processes are being rejuvenated with this miraculous, perfect, ultraviolet light. Vibrations of healing are resounding rhythmically, coursing through your energy matter, regulating and healing you.

I am breathing in and releasing my mind.

I am breathing out and releasing my mind.

I am breathing in and relaxing my body.

I am breathing out and relaxing my body.

An active body is a healthy body.
Keep it flexible with stretches and lengthening exercises.
Keep it strong with weight-bearing and core muscle strength exercises.

Your Third Eye

Once you have fully connected with your physical body, your breathing, your conscious mind, and you feel grounded in your sense of self, you can readily connect with your subconcious mind. Settle into the most comfortable position for you; seated in a chair or lying on the floor. Be open physically, palms up and open, no crossed limbs. Squared body, solid form, gentle faced. Then close your eyes and allow your conscious mind to be still. Notice the internal stimuli of your brain's energy. Thoughts, pictures, fleeting wisps of smoky light may surface in your mind's eye. Ask to speak to your higher power, your internal wisdom, your spiritual guide. See what comes to you. It could be a wise old man, a wise old woman, a golden light, Jesus Christ, God, whatever face it shows you has symbolic importance to you. It will be a kind gentle energy, never intrusive. It is at your beck and call. It can be very elusive, especially if it has been ignored or abused in the past. Treat it gently and kindly and listen to what it has to say to you. Give yourself ten minutes to sit and commune with your inner wisdom, your intuition, higher power, spiritual guide. You can speak to it and ask questions as in a normal conversation. It may respond in words, pictures, feelings or a combination there of. Your job is to trust what you are picking up. When you get it you will feel an "aha" moment when the transmitted message is crystal clear and you know what you are being told.

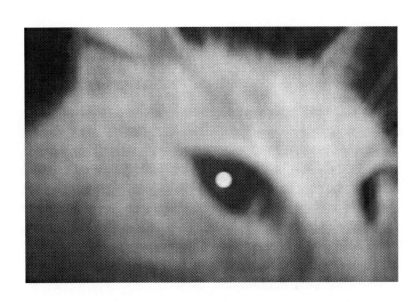

Finding Purpose

Once you have developed a trusting, stable relationship with your inner voice you can specifically ask for your purpose. It can be as monumental as saving our planet or as simple as creating a song, a piece of artwork, helping a child, or serving as an example to others of what not to be. Just kidding! Be light with your purpose, yourself, and with others. Life is an evolving joy. You can create and make of it anything that you want. My wish is for you to live with gusto, with purpose, with joy, and happiness. Give everything that you've got and trust that you will be rewarded beyond your wildest imagination, more than you could have ever thought possible.

Exercise:

- Seated comfortably on the floor or in a chair with your hands open palms facing up, with your arms and legs uncrossed, close your eyes and relax.
- Breathe deeply in and out, relax your shoulders.
- Picture yourself walking down a long, well-worn, stone staircase, you are going step by step down toward a large wooden door and the entrance to a cave.
- When you are ready open the door to the cave.
- Inside the cave you will see a flickering candle.
- Go toward the candle and settle yourself down before it on the floor of the cave.
- Ask your internal guide to come visit with you.
- Wait patiently for a sign that your guide is there with you in the cave.
- When you sense your guide is ready, ask for your purpose.
- Thank your guide.
- Leave the cave when you are ready to go.
- Gently stretch your body and open your eyes.
- You may want to write down whatever happened between you and your guide.

Exploring the Collective Unconscious

When you were connecting with your subconscious mind you might have felt a strong pull toward the collective unconscious. Carl Jung first identified the collective unconscious as being the holding place for archetypes and the inherited characteristics that all human beings share. Think of the collective unconscious as a vast interconnected web of information that exists beyond our personal minds but to which all human beings are connected.

An interesting game is to have someone you don't know any personal information about sit across from you and meditate with you. The first person thinks of someone they know and pictures them at their home. The second person then describes the images that came through to them. Then person two takes a turn. When the game works the information transmitted is amazingly accurate.

The deeper that you are able to dig below the surface of your conscious mind the better able you will be to create and find elusive answers to questions that may have long plagued you.

Be Open

Relax and open the conduits for intuition, hear your internal voice. You are an exquisite performance machine. You are everything you will ever need. All the power in the Universe is within you. Trust that what you are feeling, hearing, and intuiting is your truth. Expect that your inner truth will guide you. Expect to see miracles and magical signs in everyday life. Expect that everything will change. You will be in love with life. Listen to your intuition, your gut, your sixth sense. This is your infinite intelligence guiding your path. When you see and feel an opening act on it. Be physical, be real. Be an actor in your life. Your infinite intelligence is the producer, your conscious mind is the director, and you are the actor.

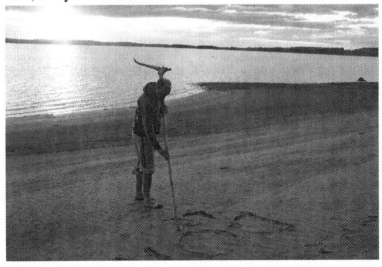

Good Advice for Bad Vices

Oh baby, you know you've got them. What they are and how they got there isn't nearly as important as how you can get rid of them. If you can stop the bad vice long enough to hear the good advice. Scary but true.

First you have to acknowledge, notice, or realize that your vice is hurting you personally. Then you have to have the desire to stop hurting yourself. Again, it comes back to knowing, loving, and seeing yourself as worthy, lovable, and valuable. Why would you hurt someone that you love and value? Why would you sabotage and destroy the hard work of a valued trusted friend? It seems the answer lies in the golden word self-esteem. Without it you've got nothing.

Humans are designed to seek pleasure, bliss feels good, the easy path, instant gratification, it all feels good. Overindulgence in alcohol, drugs, sex, food, all have a much higher price tag than you originally thought you were paying. They are addictive, self-propelling feedback loops. More is better. You have it, you crash, you need to feel good again, but you need more, more, until finally there is nothing left except you and your empty shell of comfort. It becomes unpredictable, often not satisfying, creating shame and destroying anything worthwhile that you have created.

Can you tame your vice? I believe so. Moderation in everything is the key. Balance, peace, wholeness, and solidarity with self are the goals. You have to learn to trust yourself, your boundaries, what you can and cannot do or have. Only you know what you need to do.

An exception to the idea of all things in moderation is the use of illicit drugs. Some street drugs like methamphetamines and solvents cause brain damage with a single use. These drugs batter the brain's tissue and the initial feeling of euphoria gives way to feelings of fear, terror, and paranoia. These drugs damage the brain cells that are involved in the production of feelings of pleasure and emotional control. This is a probable cause of addiction with a single use. If you are wrestling with drug addiction access every piece of information and support that you can to stop using immediately so you can halt the damage you are doing to your brain. There is emerging stem cell research that indicates nerves can rejuvenate; there is hope that if you stop soon enough you can expect new growth. An affirmation that works, "I treat my glorious brain with the respect it deserves and it's vitality and vigor is intact." Also, resolve feelings of resentment by squeezing them out with feelings of thankfulness. Feelings of resentment often lead to relapse in drug addiction.

If food is the addiction, well, isn't that beautiful? You need food to survive. You just can't use it for your every need. Treat your food with respect. Let your spirit guide you, not your emotions, when it comes to choosing and eating food. Slow down when you are eating and focus only on the food that you are eating. Pay attention to which food or food combination makes you feel fuller longer. Eat lean protein with every meal, increase your fiber intake, and increase your calcium intake. There is a hormone called leptin that suppresses appetite. Leptin is made by fat cells. Lack of sleep decreases leptin and exercise increases leptin production. That means if you exercise and sleep more your desire for food will subside.

Alcohol numbs pain, breaks down inhibitions, can make you feel stronger and less fearful. It also shuts down higher thought processes so that not only can you not create the joyful best life of your dreams, your id, your lowest impulse takes over and you are free to chaotically destroy your most cherished creations and joys. The most delicate are the first to disappear. Just remember: alcohol abuse is an unhealthy coping strategy.

"Loss of mindfulness is why people engage in useless pursuits, do not care for their own interests, and remain unalarmed in the presence of things which actually menace their welfare."
Buddha

A sexual addiction will ruin any intimate sexual relationship you have or desire to have. If you are a sex addict you are constantly obsessing about the sex act and when you can have sex again. This causes you significant distress. You are becoming increasingly secretive and you minimize your lifestyle's impact on you and those you love. You feel shame and your self-esteem is eroding. If you can work on emotionally and spiritually connecting with your partner during sexual activity you may find that your physical compulsion subsides. It will take some work for you to learn to make love from your spirit rather than your body. Try making love to your partner with your eyes open and let your spirits connect through eye contact. Look into your partner's eyes and really see the light that is within them, allow their light to enter you and nourish you.

An inability to accept dependence on others is often at the root of addiction. In order to heal you have to build self-esteem and acknowledge your need of others. When you can trust yourself you'll find that your relationships with others are trustworthy and you can depend on others.

Self-control and control of others is another tricky area around addictions. Self-esteem and self-control need to grow. Letting go of the need to control others while acknowledging that you are dependent on things that you can't control. It sounds overwhelming but it can be done.

"The more we take, the less we become."
Sarah McLaughlin, "World on Fire."

Internal Locus of Control

Exercise and Mantra

Any time that you begin a new exercise program it is important to remember that your body has limitations. So start slowly and build-up gradually according to your fitness level. If you are over forty and have not ever exercised ask your physician if you can do the physical exercises in this book. No matter what your age or fitness level you can do the cognitive exercises.

This next exercise is designed to get you under your own control. It is a cardio-vascular workout and you need to break a sweat for at least twenty minutes. You can ride a bike, jump a rope, run, use exercise equipment, speed-walk, anything that gets your heart pumping and makes you sweat. You'll have to memorize the following mantra to get the maximum benefit from this exercise. While you are exercising say the following mantra to yourself or out loud repeatedly. With each swinging motion of your body, rhythmically say the words in cadence with your movement. Focus your energy on your body's movement and your positive self- talk. So get your water bottle and start working that body!

Mantra:

I am a beloved child of the universe that created me. I love myself and I honor myself. I let others be. I am free and I am in control of myself. I love and accept myself. I am balanced. I am moderation and balance. I am perfect as I am. I am good. I am beloved. I love myself. I have everything that I need within myself. I am centered. The universe's love surrounds me and illuminates my love. I am protected.

Did you know that when you exercise to a sweat you raise your core body temperature and you kill internal viruses?

Treating Yourself with Honor and Respect

"I deserve and command respect and I will not settle for anything less. I can love without being walked over. I can have compassion without being taken advantage of."
Jon Gordon, America's #1 Energy Coach.

Your body deserves to be respected. Be gentle and good to your hair, skin, eyes, and teeth. Relax and be who you are safely and gently. Enjoy your body. Clothe yourself in warm, soft, easy fabrics that accentuate your innate glamour. Treat yourself to a massage, manicure, pedicure, or other pampering. You can pay for these services or you can do them privately and cost-efficiently at home. If you choose the latter, use whole, healthy, food products. If you can eat it you can use it topically. Extra-virgin olive oil is excellent for hair and skin. It is naturally hypoallergenic and fragrance-free. Warm a few drops in the palms of your hand and gently smooth it into your hair as a leave-in conditioner. It is also excellent as a skin moisturizer. You can use it throughout the day as a lip moisturizer and a terrific benefit is that you end up eating some of it. Olive oil is high in oleic acid and the health benefits of increased consumption of oleic acid are stunning. Your eyes and skin need the antioxidants beta carotene, vitamin C, vitamin E, and alpha lipoic acid for maximum health. Folic acid is an essential B vitamin that assists with cell division. Collagen is needed to renew body tissue. Calcium, iron, and magnesium are essential minerals that are needed for metabolism as well as tissue and bone regeneration.

Taking Time for Yourself

Depending on what stage of life you are at you will have different strategies or methods to secure the time you have to have to keep yourself well. Other people's needs are important and are definitely a consideration when deciding what your plan is to get yourself the time and space that you need to reconnect with your inner world and replenish your spirit. The time you need has to be uninterrupted. You need to know that you will have an hour or a half an hour without someone needing you. Then you can tell yourself to relax and you can really let go of the outside world and focus your attention exclusively on your inner process. Whether you are creating or meditating it really should be just you there. Trusted others can be in your space but they must be silent. No phones, pagers, radios, or children. Pets are o.k. as long as they don't disturb you.

You may need to be perfectly clear to your loved ones and tell them exactly what you are doing and that every person is not only entitled to alone time but will thrive when allowed to have it. In fact you will be better able to meet the needs of others when you meet your own needs first.

You also have to secure time to exercise your body physically. You might like to have an hour outside to go for a walk or run or two hours to go to the gym. A couple of hours to join a dance, yoga, or fitness class are your right and you can assert your right to a physically and spiritually healthy life. Conversely the others in your life are entitled to their alone time and space. With a busy family you may need to negotiate your time alone and balance it with the family's schedule. If you don't have many others in your life to organize around obviously you can choose a plan that works best for you.

You could choose early morning yoga, affirmations, meditations, and/or an evening workout.

However you can, you can make it work and you definitely deserve it.

Becoming Emotionally Wise

To be human is to feel. Emotions range in intensity, quality, and type. Some are fun, comfortable, welcome, and sought after. Others are denied, abhorred, rejected, and avoided. Emotions like anger, guilt, and jealousy are painful but we need our emotions to regulate our responses to external stimuli. It is appropriate to feel jealous when you feel the threat of loss. Someone may steal your beloved away from you. Anger motivates us to act. Guilt teaches us to do no wrong. What can happen over time though is that our emotions can begin to over-ride our common sense. What was initially used to protect us in fact destroys us. We do need to learn how to control our emotions.

Feelings make us human. We make contact with each other through our feelings. If you try to suppress any one emotion all affect is blunted. You do need to feel each and every emotion. We are tactile, emotional, watery creatures. Run your finger down your spine and you'll feel tingles throughout your body. We are electrically hard-wired to feel and we are programmed to want to feel good.

In the realm of anger, jealousy, and blame you need to let go of the desire to control others. You cannot make people do what you want them to do. They are free agents, just as you are. When you lose the need to control the outcomes, actions, thoughts, and beliefs of others you will have very little to be jealous of, angry about, or feel guilty for.

You are not in control of anything outside of your own thoughts, beliefs, and actions. You cannot control anyone else.

Anger is an emotion that feels good for some people. It is empowering, you feel larger than life, ready for action, self-righteous. Anger is an awesome emotion if you are being physically attacked and you can unleash your rage to protect yourself. However, anger is a huge problem for many people because it is extremely difficult to control. It is important to know your feelings and have conscious control over them. If you have anger under conscious control you can use it to defend yourself and others in a measured way. The Dalai Lama weighs in with his view of anger:

"Anger is the real destroyer of our good human qualities; an enemy with a weapon cannot destroy theses qualities, but anger can. Anger is our real enemy."
Dalai Lama

Fear and excitement are commingled. They are the same feeling with different cognitive attachments. Fear can keep you safe but it can also immobilize you and prevent you from acting. You can become trapped in fear. Control your fear, own it, and turn it inside out until it becomes excitement. Give it free rein and allow it to push you with an adrenalin rush outside of your safety zone.

Sadness and bereavement are normally self-limiting. They enable you to withdraw, go underground, and heal from loss. Let yourself be sad. It is o.k. to hurt. It is your pain and you own it. Hold it tight to you. The danger of sad occurs when there isn't a loss anymore and you just wallow in bereavement and self-pity. A positive feedback loop is set-up and secondary reinforcement from others enables it to continue when people pity you. Playing the victim, poor me. It is a completely self-defeating cycle.

Shame, embarrassment, and humiliation occur when your ego image of yourself is torn. There is no need for that little doillied image you have of yourself to cause such anguish. Let go of the need for others to view you as infallible. It also helps if you don't expect your idea of perfection from others.

The emotion of guilt is possibly culturally taught as opposed to being an innate emotion. Christianity teaches that people are born with original sin, leading some people to believe they are inherently bad. As well, people often use guilt to manipulate others into responding to their requests. Some positive functions of guilt are as a motivator to change and as a teacher to avoid wrongdoing. When we do wrong and feel guilty we likely won't make the same mistake again. However, when guilt becomes entrenched it inhibits emotional and spiritual growth. You feel wrong at every turn and you become immobilized. Do not live in guilt, get rid of it, dump it. If you can make amends do so if not accept that what is done is done and move on. You were doing the best you could at the time with what you knew about the situation. Try using the Serenity Prayer to handle guilt.

"God grant us the serenity to accept the things we cannot change, courage to change the things we can, and the wisdom to know the difference."
Author unknown

"Better than a thousand words is one word that gives peace."
Buddha

Music Is in You, Let it Surround You

"Music gives a soul to the universe, wings to the mind, flight to the imagination, and life to everything."
   Plato

Music affects the wave patterns in our brains and can therefore be used to alter consciousness. Throughout time various cultures have used drumming, chanting, and singing to connect with the collective unconscious, gain wisdom, and manipulate the weather.

Now that you have developed your affirmations you can begin to chant, sing, and play musical instruments to use sound vibration to impact results.

What is your song? Connecting to your internal vibration will introduce you to the music that exists within you.

Exercise and Mantra

Repeat this mantra until you feel relaxed:

I am one with the power that created me. I tune into the music in my soul. I let my music shine with the excellence that is my birthright. I am powerful, I am music, rhythm, sound, vibration, and light. My song manifests my glory.

Once you are relaxed allow any affirmation that pleases you to surface in your mind. Write it down.

Next:
Stand up tall and breathe in fully relaxing your abdomen and forcing your diaghram down with your full, complete inhalation. As you slowly exhale out, open your mouth fully and hum "ah". Let the sound vibrate up through your nose and out. This tone is high and should cause vibrations in your head. Practice breathing and humming up through your head, then dropping the "ah hum" down through your upper, then lower chest, down toward your belly button. The notes will become progressively lower. Run the sound up and down. Find the sound, tones, and vibrations that are most pleasing to you.

Finally:
Put your favorite sounds together with the words that you have chosen. Have fun with this exercise. Some people have been told that they can't sing and it is simply not true.

Mental Illness, Psychiatry, and Spirituality

Within the vast realms of mind there exists the potential for schisms between psyche, subconscious, and conscious mind. When it occurs the split causes significant cognitive impairment and is often addressed with medication. Medication acts on the neuronal synapses either inhibiting synaptic action or enhancing it. Often, and sadly, treatment with neuroleptic medication alters personality traits. It can also create physiological changes that are abhorrent to the individual. Medication is however the treatment choice for a major mental illness at this time. Schizophrenia, bipolar disorder, depression, and even personality disorders can be successfully treated with psychotropic medication. I do not think that it counters spirituality to utilize proven techniques that can enhance cognitive function. Medications could be viewed as a gift from the universe. I do believe that finding and maintaining the lowest dosage is the most life-enhancing strategy. Medication in conjunction with meditation, creativity, exercise, nutrition, and spiritual practice (cognitive affirmations) can definitely be considered a healthy treatment plan. A complete mental status examination by a trained professional can give you an accurate diagnosis. With the assistance of a licensed physician you can determine which medication can optimize your brain's chemical function.

Exercise and Mantra

I am one with the Universe that created me. I am a beloved child of the Universe and I am safe. My brain chemistry is balanced and healthy. I am intelligent, wise, and safe. My neurotransmitters and synapses are functioning perfectly.

Breathe in and out deeply and gently.

Stand upright and stretch your arms out and up. Lift up your chest as you stretch. Let your arms return gently to your sides. Take your right hand and put it on your left shoulder and take your right hand and put it on your left shoulder. Squeeze.

Embrace your divinity.

Energy Fields and Protection

You are a physical entity made up of particles and atoms that are in constant motion. The atoms are positively and negatively charged protons and ions. Basic physics. When viewed at the infinitesimal level all you are is pure molecular energy.

We exist in energy planes that consist of fluctuating impulses. There are charged spaces that we do not perceive between the atoms but that doesn't mean they don't exist. With a basic understanding of quantum physics you can imagine the energy that surrounds and suffuses you and is responsive to human thought. There is a spectrum of vibration. The lowest frequency is matter, meaning solid objects vibrate at a frequency that is perceived by the human eye. The highest frequency of vibration is thought. Thought wavelengths are attracted to wavelengths of a similar frequency.

Positive energy and negative energy are terms that have a collective meaning to us. We seek positive energy because it makes us feel good. Negative energy drains us. Nagging, bitching, griping, complaining, pessimism, all erode energy and can make a sensitive person feel under attack. You can maintain your positive energy with good nutrition, exercise, and the like already discussed but you need to protect yourself from being drained/ assaulted from the outside. Obviously environmental agents such as harsh wind, bright sun, freezing temperatures, or too hot temperatures batter our force fields. Likewise bad food, lack of sleep, or substance abuse can diminish our energy fields.

However, the biggest challenge comes from other people. Critics, pessimists, and gossips are dangerous people. You can seal your energy field from blatant negativity. Choose to be proactive with negative people and tell them the truth that their negativity drains your resources. People who judge others, who want to build hierarchies to control others often do this with gossip. It is a form of bullying that is often acceptable and sometimes seen as a form of entertainment. Shut gossip down.

We need to evolve, to grow beyond our petty egos. Embrace the gossipers and turn it around. Find something positive in what they are saying. Yes, Mary doesn't talk a lot or interact much with her co-workers. She sure knows how to enjoy silence and create a relaxing atmosphere. Don't lend an ear or a mouth to negative energy. If a person persists with the negative edge you may need to shut them out by ignoring them. It isn't your job to make everyone feel better. Just let them go in peace, and let your graceful energy heal yourself and those who embrace you.

"I am a strong and powerful force of love, compassion and strength. I will not let anyone walk through my mind with their dirty feet."
Ghandi.

Energy Healing Exercises

1. Lay on your back with your hands clasped behind your neck and your knees bent. Press the small of your back into the ground for 5-6 seconds and say to yourself, "I am grounded and one with the universe that created me."
2. Breathe deeply and relax throughout these exercises.
3. Now tuck your chin into your chest gently cradling your head in your hands and stretching the muscles in your neck stating, "I am internally blessed." Hold for 3-5 seconds and repeat two times.
4. Then press your elbows down to the floor stretching your chest upwards and state, "I love myself." Hold for 5-6 seconds. Repeat three times.
5. Stretch your right arm up and above your head and rest it on the ground stating, "I am healthy, vibrant, and secure." Hold for 8-10 seconds. Repeat with your left arm.
6. Now stand up with your feet shoulder-width apart and stretch your hands above your head gently clasping them together and state, "I consciously unify with the power and presence of the Universe within me to keep me safe and healthy." Hold for 10 seconds and repeat twice.
7. Shrug your shoulders and state, "I am relaxed." Hold for 5 seconds. Repeat twice.
8. Stretch your hands above your head, cup your left elbow in your right hand and stretch gently to the right stating, "I am blessed with forgiveness." Hold for 8-10 seconds. Repeat on your other side.

9. Clasp your hands behind your back and lean your head to the left stating, "I am flexible." Hold for 8-10 seconds. Repeat with a stretch to the right.

10. Stretch your left arm above your head, bending your arm at the elbow drop your hand behind your back, take your right hand and cup your left elbow and gently stretch your arm backward stating, "I respect myself." Hold for 15 seconds. Repeat for your right arm.

11. Take your left arm across your chest, cup your left elbow in your right hand, using your right hand pull your arm across your chest in a nice, long stretch stating, "I am strong and supple." Hold for 15-20 seconds. Repeat for your right arm.

12. Stand squarely in a doorway with your hands on each side of the doorframe at shoulder height, lean forward and state, "I know my rights and responsibilities and I take good care of myself." Hold for 15-20 seconds.

13. Bend over at your hips and stretch your arms up stating, "I am centered and in control of my force." Hold for 15-20 seconds.

14. Breathe deeply and relax.

Creating Financial Abundance

Exercise and Mantra

Money is clean. Money is abundant. Money flows easily to me. Money is my good and trusted friend. I have everything that I need. I am vastly wealthy and completely happy. The Universe that creates me ensures my financial success. I am a money magnet.

Use these affirmations and/or make up your own. Repeat them to yourself as you do the following movements:

Sit on the floor tucking your knees to your chest and hugging your knees to your chest with your arms. Tuck your chin to your chest and rest your forehead on your knees. Breathe deeply, close your eyes and say your positive money gathering affirmations. Be at peace with yourself and trust your process. Hold this position for as long as it feels good then release your body and stretch out on the floor with your arms above your head.

Repeat.

Flexibility: Mind and Body

Exercise and Mantra

1. Stand upright with your feet shoulder-width apart.
2. Relax and gently move your hips in a circular motion.
3. Continue with your hips going around and around.
4. Begin this mantra:

   I am flexible. I move with grace and ease. I see many different ways to do things. I see different angles and approaches to challenges. I am open-minded and free to see all sides of every issue. Solutions are numerous and come from many sources. I release the past.

5. Change the direction of your rotating hips.
6. Continue with the mantra.

Variations on this exercise include:

- Moving your hips in a figure 8 pattern (I like to think of it as an infinity pattern).
- Gently rolling your chin from shoulder to shoulder.

Fountain of Youth

Exercise and Mantra

Repeat the mantra in rhythmic cadence to your body's movement. Find twelve beats in the mantra that work for you and use them to count your moves.

I am youthful, sexy, healthy, radiant, energetic, and attractive. I enjoy exercising my body everyday.

I use the following 12 breaks to count:

I am youthful/sexy/healthy/radiant/energetic/and attractive/I enjoy/ exercising/my/ body/every/day/

1. Remember to breathe deeply throughout sequence.
2. Stretch your arms up above your head then bring them down to your sides.
3. Repeat 12 times.
4. Shrug your shoulders up toward your ears, relax them (drop them down).
5. Repeat 12 times.
6. Touch your toes gently stretching and rolling your spine down then

back up.
7. Repeat 12 times.
8. Put your left hand over your head and stretch to the right.
9. Repeat 12 times.
10. Put your right hand over your head and stretch to the left.
11. Repeat 12 times.
12. Do twelve squats.
13. Stand up on the balls of your feet, then down.
14. Repeat 12 times.
15. Do twelve right leg lunges.
16. Then twelve left leg lunges.
17. Do twelve push-ups.
18. Do twelve sit-ups.
19. Repeat the entire sequence at least four times.

Do this exercise every day and you will be amazed at how much younger you look and feel. For maximum benefit this should get your heart rate up, increase your respirations, and make you sweat.

One of the keys to maintaining your interest in exercising is to keep changing the program to avoid boredom. So change the exercises but keep repeating the affirmations.

For variety try working out with an exercise ball. Put on the sound of ocean waves and try push-ups, squats, and other exercises that you can safely do on a ball. You'll have fun and get a great work out.

Remember to drink water when you exercise and to breathe deeply. When you flush your body with water and oxygen you are healing yourself.

Final Thoughts

It is difficult to maintain a positive mind-set in the face of all that we experience as human beings. Personally, I have suffered significantly in my life. However, I do know that at the times that I embrace the truth of this existence, that we are spiritual beings who have control over our thoughts, emotions, and therefore our experience, I am at peace and filled with feelings of well-being and joy.

- Light is in you and flows through you
- Be open-minded
- Let go of judgement
- Create the life you want
- Find and fulfill your purpose—you are needed
- Love and approve of yourself
- Meditate
- Live in the here and now, forget the past, forgive yourself
- Change your mind, change your life
- Laughter heals
- Be yourself
- You are a beloved child of the Universe and you are free
- You are the only thinker in your head. Think nice things about yourself.
- Be open to the miracle of you and be willing to act on the opportunities that the Universe sends to you.
- Look inside and feel love, joy, and happiness
- Do less and be more
- Practice thankfulness
- Be gentle with others

Printed in the United States
58025LVS00003B/58-108